THE ULTIMATE BABY MANUAL

A Complete Guide For Parents With NewBorn Babies

Joanna Rosewood

The contents of this Book "The Ultimate Baby Manual" are derived from the personal journey and insights of the author., in partnership with her trusted midwife.

It is essential to understand that the information presented here is not intended as a substitute for professional medical advice, diagnosis, or treatment.

Rather, it serves as a reflection of one mother's experiences and the methods she learned from her trusted midwife.

Readers are encouraged to approach the content with an open mind and understand that every baby is unique, with individual needs and circumstances.

While the author shares her story and the techniques that worked for her, it is essential to recognize that what may have been effective in her situation may not necessarily apply to others.

For specific medical concerns or questions about your child's health and well-being, it is recommended to seek guidance from qualified healthcare professionals.

This book does not claim to offer comprehensive medical advice, and the author and publisher assume no responsibility for any decisions made based on the information provided herein.

By reading this book, you acknowledge and accept that the author and publisher do not guarantee the accuracy, reliability, or completeness of the information presented. The experiences shared are subjective and may not reflect the experiences or outcomes of all readers.

Ultimately, the responsibility for making informed decisions regarding the care and upbringing of your child rests with you as the parent or guardian.

This book is intended to offer support, guidance, and inspiration, but it is essential to consult with healthcare professionals and trusted advisors when making decisions that impact the health and well- being of your child.

TABLE OF CONTENTS

INTRODUCTION

As I lay in the hospital bed cradling my precious newborn in my arms, a baby boy called Leo. A whirlwind of emotions swept through me – joy, awe, pain and a huge amount of uncertainty. The exhilarating adventure of motherhood had begun. With it, the realization that I was about to embark on a journey unlike any other.

It was after midnight on the second night, it had been an exhausting day in hospital on the first. I was in labor for sixteen hours. It ended with an emergency cesarean because I couldn't naturally deliver my baby. I lay there holding Leo in my arms. Amazed by his tiny fingers and beautiful delicate features.

I knew my partner and I had no idea how to navigate each day with this tiny human. Nurses and midwives surrounded us all that day, helping with Leo. I felt clueless. What would we do when we were on our own? I felt a huge weight of responsibility. Was this going to be as easy as everyone kept telling me?

I looked down at our beautiful son. I had brought him into this world. I was going to have to raise him. We were going to have to raise him together. We had never done anything like this before. The fear of failure was overwhelming.

Did I have what it takes to be a great mom? Could I be the source of Leo's happiness and contentment? These thoughts stirred a blend of hope and nervous anticipation within me. I fell back to sleep wondering how the first night would be at home...only time would tell.

The following morning, still in the hospital, I awoke with a yearning. I wished I possessed the wealth of experience that all the skilled midwives around me had. The hospital had provided a sense of security. Which after today I would no longer have. Laying there a comforting certainty enveloped me. I knew that, upon departing the hospital, my midwife, Betty, would be there to support us once we arrived home.

I had met Betty through one of my girlfriends, a petite Greek lady. She was 63 years old and had been a midwife for over 40 years. She radiated boundless positivity. She had this unwavering confidence in handling babies. Betty was a reservoir of knowledge, simplifying every aspect leading up to labor. I clung to the hope that her reassuring touch would extend into this new chapter with Leo cradled in my arms.

In the following pages of this manual, I will share my personal journey as a new mom. I invite you to join me on a journey of discovery. Betty's tender care and profound knowledge helped shape this journey. We will navigate the intricate dance of motherhood. Merging contemporary understanding with time-honored practices.

Guided by my tiny Greek midwife Betty we will unlock the essential elements for a content baby. The Ultimate Baby Manual is what I needed when I left the hospital that day. Almost like a blueprint of what to do and when to do it. Nothing complicated, simple practices that worked for me and my two boys. Yes I made it through my first born and the second felt like a breeze.

I wrote this guide based on my experience as a new mom and what worked for me, it is not intended to be medical advice.

I have had the most amazing experience with my newborn babies. I will share this simple formula that worked for me on the following pages. The manual is not only intended for new moms but can also help moms on their second, third or fourth child. I'm confident this manual will help you as well as it did me. You too can go from zero to superhero on your journey of motherhood.

Love and light

Joanna x

CHAPTER 1

THE FIRST NIGHT DISASTER

Having said goodbye to all the amazing nurses and midwives we set off on our way home. The drive home was a strange feeling. Instead of two, there were three of us now!.

My husband usually drives like a Nascar racer. However, he transformed into a patient chauffeur like the one in "Driving Miss Daisy." We must have broken the world record for the slowest car journey home with a newborn baby. I was thankful though as I was still in pain from the birth.

As we headed home with baby Leo for his first night, the car felt cozy but kind of tired, like me. Leo, all wrapped up in his car seat, started to wake up. His little eyes opened, like when you first wake up and it's a bit bright. A tiny cry came out, like he was saying, "Hey, I'm here!" It made my heart feel super happy. It was like Leo was talking in a secret language that only moms understand.

I couldn't help thinking about how cool this first car ride was. It's the start of many adventures and firsts we'll have together as a family.

We arrived back late afternoon, Leo had fallen back to sleep in the car. It was lovely to be home.

The First Night Disaster

The journey from the hospital to our front door felt like crossing a threshold into a new world. In this world, we would be the guardians of a tiny life, our newborn son Leo.

I was so exhausted. I desperately wanted a nice, warm, relaxing bath. But I was anxious about taking one after the cesarean. So I decided to wait until Betty was here the following day.

My husband and I managed to get everything organized for the night ahead. My confidence was growing that I could do this and everything would be ok. Little did I know how the night would go.

Eager to embrace the journey of motherhood, I had already made the decision to breastfeed my baby, drawn by the beautiful bond it promised. However, the reality of breastfeeding would prove more challenging for me than the reassuring demonstrations by the midwives at the hospital.

The maternity ward was cozy and controlled. It was worlds apart from our relaxed home. We were all alone, left to our own devices, which we were about to make up as the night unfolded.

I had decided to feed Leo as late as possible that night, thinking if I was tired he must be tired. Then hoping that would be enough to get us through the night into early morning. I knew Betty was coming around first thing in the morning to check on me and Leo, which was reassuring. Just one night to get through, how bad could it be. I thought. Leo had other ideas, he had not agreed to what my plan was.

The following is a timeline of how the evening unfolded and turned into our first night disaster:

8 PM:

I was watching some TV with my husband to kill the time when Leo woke up crying.

So we did what we had learned at the hospital. We changed his diaper and then swaddled him (more on these later) and then I went about feeding him again. He latched on fairly quickly, to my relief and then started to feed. It wasn't the longest feed that we had had together in the last three days however he seemed happy and content. He fell back to sleep in my arms so I put him down in his crib next to our bed.

9:15 PM:

I carefully placed baby Leo in his crib, hoping he'd sleep soundly. The room, once filled with the soft sounds of his feeding, now embraced a stillness. I decided it was a good time to get some sleep.

As I got into bed slowly, a mixture of relief and exhaustion settled over me. The weight of motherhood, the sleepless nights, and the constant worry began to lift, if only for a moment. Watching Leo peacefully drift into slumber brought a flood of emotions—joy, gratitude, and a profound sense of love. Finally, I allowed myself to sink into the embrace of my own bed, the promise of a few precious moments of rest ahead. In that quiet space, the sweet relief of sleep awaited.

However, the peace we had hoped for quickly dissipated. Leo's cries pierced the silence, echoing off the walls, transforming the room into an arena of what would be sleepless battles.

10:15 PM:

I glanced at the clock, only one hour of sleep. How could that be? It felt like I had been asleep for hours.

In the brightly lit room (a mistake on our behalf), I moved Leo from the crib and sat in the rocking chair, desperately trying to decipher the needs of our restless baby. My husband and I exchanged glances that spoke volumes—a look of what's wrong with him. Our attempts to create a serene environment for Leo were met with relentless cries, leaving us questioning our ability to navigate the night ahead.

I wasn't sure why he had woken up. Whilst I had been in the hospital the midwives would take him at night time to let me rest and recover. So I did what I had learnt so far. I changed his diaper which was relatively dry and then went about feeding him some more milk, after all why was he awake crying. He must be hungry, I thought. This worked and he dozed off back to sleep.

11:05 PM:

After falling back to sleep relatively quickly it was again short lived. We were woken again by Leo crying, this time it was a slightly different cry. Which only a mother can instinctively tell, that secret language again. We put all the lights on again in the bedroom. This time it was clear that he had a diaper that needed changing, you could smell it!! It was only a small number two, really tiny. So after a quick change, I wrapped him up again in a swaddle and placed him back down. Turned off all the lights and we all fell back to sleep.

11:50 PM:

In the deep stillness of the night, I was stirred awake by the delicate sounds of Leo, a symphony of his suckling and unfamiliar noises. In the quiet darkness, I hesitated, thinking maybe he'd settle back into a slumber on his own. But he didn't. His soft sucking transformed into a gentle cry, escalating into a crescendo that echoed through the silence.

My husband and I stumbled out of bed, turned on all the lights and went through the same routine. We checked his diaper – nothing. So then I just instinctively decided to feed him again, he must be hungry. This time, I thought maybe a longer feeding would be the answer, though uncertainty lingered.

The time ticked away as I cradled him, an intimate dance between mother and child. As the feed extended into the night, lasting an entire hour, I grappled with the uncertainty of whether this was the right course of action. Eventually, Leo surrendered to sleep again, and with gentle hands, I swaddled him once more, returning him to the sanctuary of his crib.

The uncertainty of breastfeeding Leo would cast a shadow on my early attempts. It would leave me grappling with the delicate balance of nourishing my baby. Sometimes, it felt like he was drinking a lot, but I wasn't sure if he was getting enough.

In these moments of uncertainty, I longed for the gentle guidance of the midwives. They had made it seem effortless at the hospital. I understood that this journey into breastfeeding would be a process of learning and adapting. One which we would get to practice a lot in the coming hours.

1:20 AM:

This time, his cry echoed louder, more urgent, and my heart clenched with a mix of confusion and concern. What was bothering my precious Leo? I felt lost, with no clear answer. I scooped him up, cradling him in my arms as I sank into the rocking chair. Bouncing him in my arms to try and comfort him. Talking to him to reassure him he was safe and loved. The rocking chair became our refuge, and together, we succumbed to the gentle lullaby of sleep.

1:50 AM:

The rocking chair cradled us in a peaceful moment until Leo woke up again, crying for another meal. Tired but determined, I lifted him gently, feeling the familiar weight of his warmth. I settled into the rhythm of feeding, his hungry cries slowly turning into quiet, satisfied feeding. Or so I thought.

I was exhausted and just wanted to sleep through the night. So I could make it to the morning when I knew Betty would be round to help with everything. After Leo's feeding, I carefully placed him back into his crib, hoping he would continue his peaceful slumber.

2:30 AM:

Just 40 minutes later, his cries pierced the quiet of the room once again. The exhaustion clung to me like a heavy blanket, and my heart sank with each cry. I rushed to his side, scooping him up into my arms, feeling the warmth of his tiny body against mine. I rocked him, whispering reassurances in the hopes that he would find comfort and rest. The minutes ticked by, and as his cries gradually softened, I carefully laid back on my bed with him in my arms, praying that this time he would find the tranquility he needed. The bedroom returned to a hushed stillness as we all fell back to sleep, all three of us in bed together.

3:45 AM:

After probably our longest sleep of the night, Leo woke again once more. In the midst of these efforts, my husband, sensing the struggle, offered to take Leo for a soothing car ride. Grateful for the support, I handed over our restless little one to his father, hoping the sound of the engine would coax him into a peaceful sleep, just like on the journey home from the hospital. As the car pulled away into the quiet night, I took a deep breath, knowing that this was just another chapter in the intricate dance of parenthood.

4:15 AM:

When my husband returned from the car ride, a wave of relief washed over me as I saw Leo sound asleep in his car seat. The gentle rise and fall of his chest brought a sense of calm to the room, and I couldn't bear to disturb him.

Exhaustion hung heavy in the air, but there was a shared understanding between my husband and me. Rather than risk waking Leo, we carefully left him in the car seat, nestled and cocooned in the serenity of dreams. In that quiet moment, the hope for a precious hour of uninterrupted sleep became our lifeline, a collective wish to just make it through the rest of the night.

As we retreated to our bed, I couldn't help but marvel at the resilience of parenthood—the ability to find solace in the small victories and the enduring strength that comes from facing the challenges together as a family.

6:00AM

As we stirred from our brief respite, I couldn't help but reflect on the night that had unfolded— the cries, the struggles with feeding, and the impromptu car ride. It felt like a complete disaster in my eyes, a chaotic initiation into the unpredictability of parenthood.

Yet, as I looked at my husband and our peacefully sleeping Leo, there was a shared sense of accomplishment. We had weathered the storm together, emerging on the other side with a newfound strength.

The challenges of that first night at home had etched themselves into the narrative of our parenthood journey, a testament to the resilience that comes from facing the unknown with love, patience, and a willingness to embrace the imperfect beauty of family life.

CHAPTER 2
AN ANGEL ARRIVES

It's our first morning together at home and there is a knock at the door. The one that I have been secretly waiting for.

It's Betty, our seasoned Greek midwife arriving at our doorstep like a beacon of hope. Her arrival marked the beginning of a new chapter in our parenthood journey. This chapter unfolded with both expertise and unexpected hilarity. Her presence exuded a calming assurance. It immediately puts my anxious mind at rest.

As she stepped into our chaotic household, Betty sensed our fatigue. She immediately orchestrated a well-needed oasis- a soothing bath to ease the exhaustion.

I immersed myself in the warm water. Betty, a seasoned caregiver, delicately washed away the weariness of the night. She tended to my Cesarean wound with gentle hands. She redressed it with a tenderness that spoke volumes of her vast experience.

Then with a knowing smile, she dove into the heart of the matter. She listened as I poured out the tale of the previous night's disaster.

An Angel Arrives

I told her about my struggles with breastfeeding, the endless cries, and the feeling of helplessness. With wisdom cultivated over 40 years, Betty embraces my despair with an air of authority and warmth. In the blink of an eye, she took charge, turning our chaotic home into one of reassurance.

Her gentle guidance and soothing words transformed the narrative from one of despair to hope. Instilling a sense of confidence in both of us as new parents. As Betty worked her magic, I felt the weight of the night's uncertainties lifting. The comforting knowledge that we were in the capable hands of a true angel of motherhood replaced me.

Betty's gentle yet authoritative Greek tone reassured me. She said that breastfeeding was a skill. It required practice, patience, and a sprinkle of wisdom. Leo, with his tiny hands and eager appetite, became her willing pupil.

Yet, as she guided me through the nuances of breastfeeding, a furrow appeared on her brow. With a keen observation, Betty recognized that my nipples weren't releasing enough milk. This revelation explained the baby's cries through the night.

"Why darling," she proclaimed. "No wonder Prince Leo is crying, he is starving" Only Betty would call him Prince Leo. She was never fazed by his crying. She would always say it was his only way of talking. How else would he let us know something was wrong?

With compassion, she assured me that this was a common challenge. She offered guidance on addressing it. She suggested a shift to bottle feeding using formula milk Recognizing that my struggle with breastfeeding would impact both my well-being and the baby's nourishment.

At first, the idea stirred a mix of emotions within me: guilt, disappointment, and a sense of failure. Betty offered comforting guidance. She explained that the priority was ensuring the baby received adequate nourishment. She added that bottle feeding offered a practical solution.

As we made the transition, I began to understand that this decision wasn't a concession. It was a thoughtful choice to focus on my baby's well-being. The bottle became a vessel of love. It guaranteed that each feeding time was a comforting moment for my little one.

Betty's support made shifting from breastfeeding to bottle feeding a liberating choice. It freed me from guilt and it would let me enjoy watching my baby thrive with each contented gulp.

Meanwhile, my husband, a towering man, found himself at the mercy of this tiny powerhouse. Betty had him scurrying around like a tornado under her command. He fetched bottles, clothes, blankets, towels, and swaddles. He also prepared herbal teas and whatnot.

She had him dancing to her merry little Greek tune. It was like a hilarious dance routine, and I swear he must have hit his 10,000 steps during Betty's first visit.. Every time she issued a new order, his sheepish grin would imply, "Betty, you're the boss!" But the kicker? Every command she gave him came with a cheeky wink from her in my direction.

My husband wore a sheepish grin and thought he was the hero of the day, oblivious to the puppeteering at play. Little did he know that grin was Betty's creation. It was a masterpiece of mischievous puppet mastery. It left me smiling at the ongoing comedy show unfolding in our bedroom.

Prince Leo as Betty insisted on calling him, in his own intuitive way, seemed to sense the arrival of this seasoned midwife, as if a comforting aura surrounded her. As she took charge with her gentle but authoritative manner, Leo's eyes sparkled with a curious anticipation.

It was as if he knew that the caring hands that had cradled generations were now turning their attention to him. Betty, with her decades of experience, prepared Leo for his first bath. His tiny fingers wrapped around her seasoned ones. This created a silent bond between them.

The moment Betty lowered Leo into the small plastic baby bath felt like an initiation into a world of firsts. The unfamiliar sensation startled Leo. He let out a series of loud screams that echoed through the room. New screams that I had not yet heard from him. Yet, in Betty's expert hands, those initial screams morphed into a soothing melody of calm.

As she poured warm water over him, Leo's tensed body relaxed. He surrendered to the gentle caress of the bath. The room was once filled with the sharp notes of cries. Now, it resonated with the soothing sounds of water. Betty's voice reassured Leo what a good boy he was during his first ever bath at home.

After the bath, Betty unveiled another cherished tradition. She gave my adorable baby boy a gentle full-body massage, using baby-friendly massage oil. Betty wisely recommended waiting until the baby reaches at least two weeks of age before incorporating this into every bath time. In the present moment, it served as another insightful demonstration from her to us.

The fragrance of the oil filled the air, creating a sensory experience. Betty, with her nimble fingers, massaged Leo's delicate skin in a dance of love and tradition. The rhythmic strokes seemed to lull him into a state of serene bliss. It was as if the oil carried not just the wisdom of the ancients, but also the promise of well-being and connection.

After the relaxing bath, Betty dresses Leo for bed and holds him in her experienced arms. She confidently gives him the bottle, moving in a smooth, dance-like way. While Leo drinks, the room is filled with a peaceful and quiet feeling. Betty, with a knowing smile, demonstrates the art of winding—the crucial ritual to ensuring a happy and comfortable baby.

I confessed to being too gentle in my previous attempts at patting the baby's back. Betty, with her trademark firmness, took charge. She positioned Leo against her shoulder. She demonstrated a purposeful patting technique. It sent vibrations through Leo's tiny back.

She then sits him on her lap and supports his tiny head under his chin. She rubs and pats his back. I won't say it's forceful. Betty uses a confident technique. This allows Leo to release a gentle but strong burp.. This signals the successful release of wind, ensuring he's comfortable and content.

In that moment, the room became a classroom of parenthood. The seasoned instructor, Betty, imparted invaluable lessons with a touch of firmness and a sprinkle of humor. We were both grateful for the guidance. We realized that sometimes, a bit of confident patting is exactly what's needed to coax out a contented burp from a well-fed baby.

In the presence of Betty, Leo seemed to sense he had met his match in the realm of soothing magic. She expertly wrapped him in a snug swaddle. He surrendered to the cocoon of warmth, his tiny body embraced like a secure secret. Betty's swaddle worked like magic, a captivating hug that eased him into a peaceful sleep.

Placed gently into his crib, Leo's eyes fluttered slowly, as if to say thank you to this amazing guardian angel. Betty smiled knowingly. She assured us that he would sleep peacefully for a good few hours before the next feeding.

At that moment, as a new mother, I couldn't help but marvel at Betty's magical touch. A blend of expertise and a sprinkle of grandmotherly charm had transformed our chaotic bedroom into a haven of tranquility.

Betty, with her ever-practical approach, turned to my husband. She requested him to fetch a pen and paper. As he scrambled to find the necessary tools, Betty began outlining a meticulous routine for the rest of the day. Her words wove a tapestry of wisdom, blending practicality with a touch of timeless care.

Each step, from feeding times to nap schedules, became the foundation of a blissful and peaceful routine for baby Leo. With pen in hand, my husband wrote down Betty's instructions.

Both of us realized that these simple yet profound guidelines would become the roadmap for our days. They would offer structure and harmony in the midst of the unpredictable days of early parenthood. At that moment, as I saw the step by step plan on paper, I felt grateful for the expert guidance that had entered our lives. It set the stage for a peaceful and contented journey moving forward with our little one, Leo.

As Betty worked her magic, weaving spells of comfort and wisdom. Our home transformed into a symphony of love, laughter, and learning. Leo, now fed and content, slept in agreement, blissfully unaware of the circus that had unfolded around him. Betty, with her ageless charm and boundless knowledge, not only mended the struggles of the night. She also brought a renewed sense of confidence and joy to our new family.

In the end, our bedroom that had been a stage for a comedy of errors turned into one of triumphs. Betty, the star of the show, left us with a sleeping and content baby and a trove of memories and newfound skills. That second night at home would be worlds away from our first, no pun intended but it was literally like night and day for us. Betty's formula laid out in the chapter 'The Ultimate Guide" was what we both needed.

As she bid us farewell, I couldn't help but marvel at the angelic touch she had brought to our lives. Betty, the tiny powerhouse, had not just eased our troubles. She had also become an enduring character in the tale of our parenthood journey. She left us with the gift of laughter, learning, and the promise of many more adventures to come.

CHAPTER 3

5 REASONS WHY BABIES CRY

For new moms, deciphering the cries of your baby is like unraveling a complex puzzle.

Babies communicate through crying. Understanding the specific reasons behind those cries has proven quite challenging. Delving into the various triggers that prompt these tears is crucial. It demystifies baby communication. It opens the door to a more responsive and nurturing approach to looking after them.

Remember you are learning a new language with your new born baby. Here are five common reasons why our little ones shed those precious tears.

Hungry:

Betty often emphasized that hunger was a primary culprit behind those heart-wrenching cries. "Dear," she'd say with a gentle nod, "a baby's tummy is as tiny as a pea, and it fills up fast. They'll let you know when it's time to refuel."

Her advice was simple but profound. Listen for the cues, watch for rooting or sucking motions, and ensure timely feedings.

Diaper Needs Changing:

As Betty demonstrated diaper-changing techniques, she said, "Imagine sitting in a wet or soiled diaper, dear. Not pleasant, is it? Babies feel the same way."

Her practical approach to changing diapers became a crucial part of our daily routine. It ensured Leo's comfort and curbed unnecessary cries.

Tiredness:

"Even the tiniest humans need their beauty sleep," Betty would say with a twinkle in her eye.

She urged us to observe Leo's subtle cues of drowsiness. She emphasized that over tiredness often led to fussiness. Establishing a consistent sleep routine, she taught, was key to keeping cries at bay.

Wind and tummy troubles:

Betty's wealth of experience unveiled the mysteries of a gassy tummy.

"Babies, bless their hearts, struggle to release gas," she explained. "Firm pats and massages can make all the difference."

With Betty's guidance, we learned the art of burping and soothing techniques. This ensured Leo's tummy troubles were swiftly addressed.

Including the poo technique discussed later in the book

Overstimulation:

"Babies may be small, but their senses are mighty," Betty mused. She cautioned against overwhelming environments, urging for a balanced atmosphere. "Bright lights, big groups of people—these can all be too much for a little one."

Betty often advised against tiptoeing around babies in an attempt to maintain silence.

"Let them experience the hum of everyday life," she'd say. "Being too quiet might make them too sensitive to noise. A gentle, consistent noise level is better than absolute silence. It's about finding the right balance. The baby can sleep peacefully amidst the world's natural sounds."

Betty's wisdom encouraged us to embrace a more natural soundscape. It steered us away from excessive quietness and helped Leo adapt to the ambient sounds of our home.

Betty's words were not just practical guidance but a beacon of reassurance. She reminded us that decoding cries was a nuanced art, an art of observation and response. "Each cry is a language, a way your baby communicates with you," she'd say. Her eyes reflected decades of nurturing wisdom. "Learn to listen, and you'll find the melody that soothes each one."

New parents must remember that crying is a natural part of infant communication. It doesn't always mean a problem. Pay attention to the baby's cues. Respond promptly. Seek support when needed. This can create a supportive environment for both the baby and you.

With Betty's patient guidance, we learned to interpret these different cries with newfound confidence. The house was once filled with Leo's cries. Now, it's a space for us to understand, respond, and nurture our precious little one, with every wail.

CHAPTER 4
THE ULTIMATE GUIDE

This chapter is called "The Ultimate Guide." It is a blueprint crafted from the invaluable lessons Betty bestowed upon us. It encapsulates the essence of years of her experience and my own experiences with Leo. I made small changes here and there to suit my little one. Remember, each of our babies are unique and individual. Tailor these suggestions to suit your baby's needs.

Use this guide as a practical roadmap for navigating the intricacies of baby care. Join me as we delve into the heart of this guide. We'll explore tried-and-tested methods that Betty shared with us. These insights have shaped my understanding. They've become the pillars of my parenting journey.

The Sleeping and Feeding Routine:

Drawing from her wealth of experience, Betty suggested a structured routine. It's like a gentle melody flowing through the day. She suggested specific times: 6 am (wake up), 10 am, 2 pm, 6 pm, 10 pm, and 2 am (the dream feed).

This structured approach established a sense of predictability for Leo. It empowered me to be the orchestrator of these crucial moments. Instead of Leo dictating when to feed him, I installed a routine that we both needed. This was the foundation for what would become a structured and calm day, everyday.

Following this routine became a soothing anchor. Every clock hour held a purpose, a quiet cue to attend to Leo's needs. Betty emphasized the importance of not only feeding, but also incorporating an automatic nappy change during these scheduled moments.

6:00 am:

At 6 am, the world stirred gently to life, and with it, Leo's morning routine unfolded. Waking Leo with a tender touch, the first order of the day was a diaper change. It was a gradual introduction to the waking world. Fresh clothes replaced the cozy warmth of his swaddle, setting the tone for the day that lay ahead. Next job preparing his feed

When the feed was ready, I would swaddle him as Betty showed me (more on this later). Then, I would feed him and wind him. This usually took one hour.

I would always make sure to leave a small amount of milk in the bottle when winding Leo. I'd use this last drop of milk to help him doze off back to sleep at the end of the feed once he had been properly winded. Just as Betty had demonstrated the first day.

This whole process of waking, changing his diaper, clothes and then feeding would take roughly one and a half hours. At the start of our journey together some days would take a little longer. As I grew in confidence with Leo and the routine over the coming days and weeks it would take less time.

I would then place him in his crib to sleep, wrapped all nice and snug in his swaddle

10 am and 2 pm:

Sometimes he would already be awake, other times he would be sound asleep. Regardless, at 10am and 2pm, I would wake him up and use the same process I used for the first feed at 6am.

This way, I could structure my day and get all the other bits and pieces done that I needed to do. I knew he would be sleeping until the times we had set using this routine.

6 pm and 10pm - Including bathtime.

This would be the evening routine we would use for our two boys for the years to come. Dinner, then bath time, then bedtime.

The key here was waking Leo up at 6pm for supper and then in the bath every night at 8pm.

Using the time after the bath to get him ready for bed and his 10pm feed.

At 6pm it would be the same routine as the 6am, 10am, and 2pm feeding times. Diaper change, then feeding.

At 8 pm, it signaled the commencement of Leo's nightly bath. The warm water would always welcome him. Bath time was like a special ritual for all of us. Bath time wasn't about only getting him clean; it was a peaceful break in our day, a time for us to bond and have fun together.

After his bath, Leo received a full-body massage. The tender touch became a cherished tradition. The soothing strokes and gentle kneading after the bath enhanced our bond. They also added relaxation to his bedtime routine.

After the bath and massage, we headed upstairs to our quiet, dimly lit bedroom. This was our peaceful space, away from the noise downstairs. Here Leo could settle down before his 10 pm feed.

Sometimes, the feed happened right on time, and other times, it was a little earlier. Keeping Leo awake between feeds and adding the bath made sure he was ready for bed after his 10 pm bottle.

The 10 pm feed was like a comforting lullaby, happening quietly in our bedroom. The low-stimulus environment ensured a gentle transition to sleep.

As I placed him down to rest, the 6 pm to 10 pm schedule became more than a routine. It was a sequence of curated moments preparing him for bedtime. They whispered calm lullabies to our little one. They invited him into the tranquil embrace of a night's sleep.

2am - The dream feed

The 2 am feeding, or as Betty called it "the dream feed," was a strategic and gentle approach. Its goal was to cut disruption to both Leo's sleep and our well-deserved rest.

In a softly lit room, the feeding takes place. There is a deliberate intention to keep stimulation to a minimum.

We would check the diaper here to see if it needed changing, and if it was still dry, we would not change it. Only changing when necessary in the middle of the night. So not to stimulate Leo too much.

Only the sound of the kettle boiling would break the silence of the room as we prepared to warm up the milk. Then after a re-swaddle, feeding would begin. Making sure to wind him properly. Then, another re-wrap of the swaddle and back down to sleep. On a good night this would take 45 mins. The longer dream feeds required more winding as well as a diaper change.

The dream feed serves a dual purpose.

First, it allows the baby to receive nourishment without fully waking up. This enables a smoother transition back to sleep.

Secondly, incorporating this feeding into the night helps extend the duration between nighttime wake-ups. This contributes to longer stretches of uninterrupted sleep for both the baby and the parents.

The key to the success of the dream feed lies in its simplicity. The parent refrains from engaging the baby in conversation or unnecessary stimulation. Diaper changes are made with minimal disruption. Ensuring that the whole process is swift and conducive to a quick return to the land of dreams.

When I started, I was skeptical about this routine's effectiveness. Yet, the guidance of Betty, coupled with the disaster of our first night, prompted me to embrace it.

Our first attempt at the dream feed was in stark contrast to the chaos of our first night. It worked like a dream (no pun intended).

In that moment, the room transformed from a battleground of cries and confusion on that first night into a sanctuary of quiet joy.

Although I never got used to waking up in the middle of the night to carry out these feeds (who does right?) It was rewarding knowing that Leo received the nourishment that he needed without fully waking. So we, in turn, could get some well needed sleep.

"For many years, I've seen the power of a well-crafted routine," Betty shared with a twinkle in her eye. "By waking the baby on these scheduled hours, we instill a sense of rhythm. By guiding the child into a pattern that aligns with their natural biological clock. This way, moms and dads assume control over the feeding schedule. They nurture a routine. This routine ensures everyone finds peace in the predictability of these precious moments."

Waking my little one every four hours seemed counterintuitive at first. Still, as I saw the magic unfold, I became a fervent believer in the power of this routine. At first, the wake-up calls were hard. Yet, they became a peaceful routine of feeding, soothing, and back to sleep. This gave us both structure and reassurance.

By adhering to these scheduled hours, a profound transformation occurred. Leo adapted to the predictability. As parents, we found ourselves gaining precious hours of undisturbed sleep. The 6 am awakening became a gentle greeting, setting the tone for a day filled with nourishment and rest.

As the days turned into weeks, and weeks into months. The sleep and feeding routine became cherished in our lives. The structured hours emerged as a reliable anchor in the unpredictable journey of parenthood.

Thanks to Betty's timeless wisdom and the implementation of this routine, we all found comfort in this simple but effective roadmap that guided us through each new day together.

Swaddling:

Swaddling became one of my secret weapons with Leo.

It was like wrapping him in a warm, comforting hug that whispers, "You're safe, you're loved." Thanks to Betty, I learned that swaddling gave my baby a sense of security, like creating a cocoon of comfort. It's not just about routine; it's a ritual filled with love and care.

As I gently wrapped him, I felt his tension melting away. Swaddling created a safe space for my precious one to rest peacefully. A simple act that makes a world of difference in ensuring a calm, cozy, and restful sleep for my little bundle of joy.

There were four reasons why Betty had been doing this for years. She would say that number one it gives babies a sense of security. It makes them feel cozy and safe, almost like being back in the tummy.

Swaddling also helps with something called Startle Reflexes. These reflexes are involuntary movements in their arms and legs. They happen until they get older and learn to control them. These movements are involuntary. Babies are often startled by them. This can affect their sleep.

Swaddling their arms limits big movements. For that reason, they are less likely to be startled and wake up when sleeping.

Swaddling helps maintain the baby's back-sleeping position. It also reminds parents to place the baby on its back to sleep, which is considered the safest sleeping position at the newborn stage. Lastly, It's like wrapping them in a warm blanket that keeps them just right—neither too hot nor too cold.

Swaddling is not just a bedtime routine. It's like a superpower blanket that gives babies a sense of security, stops surprise jumps, keeps them safe, and makes sure they're cozy and at the right temperature. I learnt from Betty and our own experience that swaddling is a fantastic way to make sure Leo slept soundly and happily.

Water:

This was another one of Betty's little tricks.

She shared an unorthodox but surprisingly effective tip for those early wake-ups with my newborn. Suggesting we offer a little water (about 5oz) mixed with half a teaspoon of brown sugar. This would be made fresh everyday, with boiled water and cooled down in the fridge.

At first, it sounded unconventional, but Betty assured me it would work like a charm. Her reasoning was simple yet intriguing. We, as humans, are made up of water. So, a gentle sip might tide over his hunger until the proper feeding hour.

Skeptical yet curious, I tried this method during those unexpected early awakenings. They usually happened about an hour before his scheduled feed. To my surprise, it proved to be the perfect solution. It offered a soothing and temporary remedy until the next scheduled feeding session.

Of course, Betty's advice worked wonders for me and both of my boys, but I understand that every baby is different. New moms, I would emphasize the importance of consulting with your own midwife or GP before trying this advice.

Every baby has unique needs, and what worked for one might not be suitable for another. Prioritize the baby's health and well-being. Seek professional guidance to make sure unconventional methods fit individual circumstances. Betty's wisdom was a valuable addition to my parenting journey. I'd encourage others to consider it and research it. After all, it made sense to me to give my baby water as well as the milk.

The Poo Technique:

Betty unveiled a unique technique as her secret weapon for easing babies' bowel movements. As she would say, not all newborn babies, but some, needed help with their number two's. Leo fell into the camp of the ones that did.

She demonstrated how laying the baby on its back and drawing both legs back toward its head, exposing the tiny bottom would help him pass his number two. Armed with a cotton wool pad soaked in warm/hot water, the method involved applying gentle pressure in a downward stroking motion on the baby's bum. This approach aimed to stimulate the natural reflexes that encourage bowel movements.

"It may sound unconventional," Betty assured me, "but this method can be quite effective. It can provide relief for the baby and promote regular bowel habits." She would go on to say that if the newborn baby struggles with passing their number two's then the constant feeding would make them feel like a stuffed little piggy. Helping them to push out their number two's would be a relief for them to take on more feed. As a guide we would use how hard Leo's tummy felt and also note in our mind if he had not had a poo in the last 12 hours.

The more Betty demonstrated this on her visits, the more we tried this on our own. I was amazed at how easily Betty made this work. It was like watching soft whip ice cream pour out from Leo's bum when Betty would take control. Over time, both my husband and I perfected this technique, ensuring regular bowel movements for our little one.

As with any advice, you should consult with healthcare professionals to ensure the technique aligns with the baby's individual needs and health considerations.

Dummy or no dummy:

The question of whether newborn babies should have a pacifier, or dummy, is a matter of personal choice for parents.

Some argue that pacifiers can offer comfort to a fussy baby and help with self-soothing. They also argue that using pacifiers during naps or bedtime may reduce the risk of sudden infant death syndrome (SIDS).

On the other hand, opponents of pacifier use worry about potential dental issues. They are also concerned about interference with breastfeeding and dependence issues.

As a new parent, you must weigh the potential benefits and drawbacks. Consider the baby's individual needs. Then, consult with healthcare professionals for personalized advice. Ultimately, the choice to introduce a dummy to a newborn rests with you. As only you can make an informed decision based on your baby's comfort and well-being.

Betty, our trusted midwife, had a unique perspective on this matter. She believed that if we followed the feeding and sleep routine diligently, there might not be a need for a pacifier. According to her, a consistent routine provided babies with a sense of security and comfort. This reduced the need for additional soothing methods.

Betty encouraged us to try and avoid using pacifiers. Instead, she suggested creating a nurturing environment. This would promote natural sleep patterns and self-soothing techniques. The philosophy was rooted in simplicity. It trusted in our baby's innate abilities to find comfort and contentment with the routine that we would deliver.

Smiling or winded:

Betty often dispels the common myth surrounding smiling babies. They may actually be suffering from trapped wind after feeding. She emphasized that smiles in newborns are not always signs of joy. They can also indicate discomfort caused by unexpelled gas.

From Betty's perspective, recognizing the signs of a baby needing to burp involves observing cues such as squirming, restlessness, and the baby pulling away from the breast or bottle mid-feed. These subtle signs may indicate the presence of trapped air that needs to be released.

As a mother, learning to decode these cues became crucial in understanding Leo's needs. Betty guided me in the art of burping. She encouraged firm patting on the baby's back after each feed to ensure any trapped air found its way out. This simple yet vital practice has proven effective in minimizing my baby's discomfort. It also ensures that those adorable smiles are indeed expressions of joy rather than signs of hidden discomfort.

Babies start to smile naturally between six to eight weeks of age. This timeframe aligns with their developmental milestones. They become more aware of their surroundings and responsive to stimuli.

Around this age, you may notice your baby's first social smiles. These are not just reflexes, but also deliberate and responsive to external stimuli, such as your face or voice. It's important to differentiate between these social smiles and the reflexive smiles that newborns often exhibit in their sleep.

As a mother, I find it fascinating and rewarding to recognize the timing of these developmental milestones. It marks the beginning of more interactive and emotionally expressive moments with my growing baby.

Diaper changing:

Betty bestowed upon me a valuable lesson in the art of diaper changing. It transcended the mere act itself. With experience, she demonstrated the technicalities. She also showed the essence of confidence in this routine task.

As a mother, I learned that the key was to convey a sense of assurance to my baby. I let them know that I was in control and they had nothing to fear. Betty emphasized the importance of maintaining eye contact. She also stressed speaking soothingly and using gentle yet deliberate movements. She highlighted that this seemingly mundane task was an opportunity to build trust and establish a secure connection with my baby.

As I adopted Betty's guidance, diaper changes transformed into moments of bonding, fostering a sense of security for my little one. The reassurance I provided during these moments echoed Betty's wisdom. It reminded us that even simple tasks can be meaningful moments between parent and child.

Bathtime and massage:

Bath time became a cherished ritual. It wasn't just for cleanliness. It was an opportunity for my newborn baby and me to unwind and enjoy precious moments together. Betty shared invaluable insights on making bath time a calming experience. She emphasized the significance of pouring water carefully over the baby's head. She quoted, "Gentle streams of water, like soft whispers, help them feel secure.""

With each bath, I learned to create a soothing ambiance. I used warm water and calming words to reassure my baby. Betty's wisdom echoed in my ears as I cradled my little one. I ensured that every splash was a gentle embrace, not a surprise. Bath time transformed into a serene occasion. It was a chance for my baby to relax and for me to savor these tender moments of bonding.

Betty's guidance shaped the practicalities of bath time. It also added a touch of wisdom. This turned this routine into a cherished experience. It nurtured the special connection between my baby and me.

Betty offered wise advice for holding my baby during bath time. She made sure the environment was safe and secure. With gentle confidence, she demonstrated the ideal technique – supporting their delicate head with my forearm, whilst interlocking my thumb and index finger around Leo's armpit. "A secure hold is like a comforting hug," she would say.

I adopted the method Betty shared, establishing a firm yet gentle grip. This technique not only offered physical support but conveyed a sense of reassurance to my little one.

I held my baby close, following Betty's wisdom. Bath time became a haven of tranquility, fostering trust and enhancing the bond between us. The simple act of holding, guided by Betty's expert advice, transformed routine bath times into cherished moments of connection and security for both me and Leo.

The massage after bath time emerged as a delightful tradition, adding an extra layer of connection and relaxation for both my little one and me. Betty, with her wealth of experience, introduced me to the soothing benefits of using baby massage oil, turning this routine into a cherished moment of tenderness.

As I gently massaged Leo's tiny limbs, I observed a visible delight on his face. A symphony of content coos and fluttering eyelashes signaling his enjoyment. Betty often compared it to how adults feel rejuvenated after a full-body massage. The same principle applied to babies.

This pre-bedtime ritual wasn't just about physical relaxation. It was also a holistic approach to preparing my baby for sleep. The rhythmic strokes and the fragrant baby massage oil created a serene atmosphere. This calmed my baby's senses and set the stage for a peaceful night ahead.

As I continued this practice, it became a cherished part of our bedtime routine. It fostered a sense of security and tranquility. This led to more restful nights for both of us. Betty's wisdom enhanced the practical aspects of caregiving. It also infused our daily routines with warmth and connection, making the journey of parenthood truly special.

Rocking or bouncing:

Rocking or bouncing newborn babies can have both positive and negative effects.

Gentle rocking or bouncing motions can soothe a fussy baby. They can also help them fall asleep by mimicking the rhythmic movements they experienced in the womb. This can provide comfort and security to the baby. It helps regulate their emotions and promote relaxation.

However, excessive rocking or bouncing may lead to overstimulation or dependence on motion for sleep. This makes it challenging for the baby to settle without constant movement. Additionally, prolonged rocking or bouncing can contribute to motion sickness in some babies.

As a mother, I've found myself grappling with the idea of rocking or bouncing my newborn baby. On one hand, it's a soothing technique that seems to calm most babies and lull them into peaceful sleep. However, Betty was adamant about the drawbacks of such a practice. "It's fine when they're a few weeks old," she'd say. "But what happens when they're almost a year old, bigger, heavier, and have become used to rocking and bouncing?""

Betty's words echoed in my mind, reminding me to consider the long-term implications. While the immediate comfort of rocking or bouncing may seem appealing. The downside was creating a dependency that could prove challenging to break as the baby grows. Balancing the pros and cons was a dilemma I grappled with. Betty's wisdom guided me in making informed decisions for the well-being of my baby.

In the end, my husband and I decided not to rock or bounce our baby boys. We followed Betty's advice and trusted our own instincts as parents.

It wasn't always easy. Relatives or friends would eagerly offer to hold Leo and instinctively start rocking or bouncing him. However, we politely explained that we preferred not to use those techniques. We emphasized Betty's expert guidance and our commitment to consistency. It was a conscious choice. It required patience and persistence. We believed it was in the best interest of our babies' long-term sleep habits and overall development.

Reflecting on our journey, I realized that many parents may default to rocking or bouncing. They do this simply because it's a common practice they've observed in others. However, by trusting in our own instincts and seeking guidance from trusted sources, we were able to chart a path that felt right for our family.

CHAPTER 5

THE ESSENTIALS

Preparing for the arrival of a new baby is an exciting yet overwhelming journey. As expecting parents, it's important to ensure that you have all the essential items ready. This will help welcome your little one into the world. This comprehensive list contains essentials for every parent to consider purchasing before their baby arrives. It includes practical necessities and comforting comforts.

1. Crib or Bassinet:

A safe and comfortable sleeping space for your baby is paramount. Whether you choose a crib or bassinet, make sure it meets safety standards. Also, make sure it provides a cozy environment for your little one to rest.

2. Baby Clothes:

Stock up on onesies, sleepers, socks, hats, and other clothing essentials. Get them in various sizes. Opt for soft, breathable fabrics that will keep your baby comfortable day and night.

3. Diapers and Wipes:

Be prepared for countless diaper changes. Stock up on diapers and wipes in different sizes.

Consider eco-friendly options if possible. Don't forget diaper rash cream to soothe your baby's delicate skin.

4. Feeding Supplies:

Whether you choose to breastfeed or formula-feed, having the right supplies is essential. Invest in a breast pump, bottles, and nipples. If needed, buy formula. Also, get nursing pads and a feeding pillow for added support.

5. Car Seat:

A car seat is essential for bringing your baby home from the hospital. It is also necessary for safe travel thereafter. Make sure it's installed correctly. Also, make sure it meets safety standards for your baby's age and weight.

6. Stroller or Baby Carrier:

For outings and adventures with your little one, a stroller or baby carrier is indispensable. Choose a model that suits your lifestyle. It should offer comfort and convenience for both you and your baby.

7. Baby Bath Tub and Toiletries:

Keep your baby squeaky clean with a baby bath tub, gentle baby soap, shampoo, and lotion. Opt for tear-free formulas to ensure a pleasant bath time experience. We steered clear of Johnson and Johnson products and used a natural baby oil for the post bath massage

8. Swaddle Blankets and Sleep Sacks:

Swaddling can help soothe your baby and promote better sleep. Stock up on swaddle blankets and sleep sacks to keep your little one snug and secure.

9. Baby Monitor:

A baby monitor provides peace of mind by allowing you to keep an eye (and ear) on your baby while they sleep. Choose a model with video and audio capabilities for added reassurance.

10. Nursery Essentials:

Create a cozy and functional nursery for your baby. Include essentials like a changing table, diaper pail, rocking chair or glider, and storage solutions for diapers, clothes, and other items.

11. First Aid Kit:

Be prepared for minor mishaps. Have a well-stocked first aid kit with all the essentials.

12. Books and Toys:

Stimulate your baby's senses and encourage development with age-appropriate books and toys. Choose options that are safe, engaging, and suitable for your baby's stage of development.

13. Parenting Books and Resources:

Invest in parenting books and resources that cover topics like newborn care, breastfeeding, sleep training, and child development. Arm yourself with knowledge and guidance. Gain as much knowledge as you can. The Ultimate Guide is a great foundation to work from.

Ensure you have these essentials on hand before your baby arrives. You'll be better prepared to navigate the joys and challenges of parenthood with confidence and peace of mind. Remember, every baby is unique. Trust your instincts and don't hesitate to seek support from healthcare professionals, family, and friends along the way.

CHAPTER 6
CLOSING THOUGHTS

From One Superhero to Another...

As I reach the final pages of this book, I'm reminded of the incredible journey that awaits every new mom who picks up these pages. It's a journey filled with ups and downs, triumphs, and challenges. Above all, it transforms us into the superheroes our little ones need.

Reflecting on my own experience, I can't help but feel grateful for the wisdom and guidance of Betty, our beloved Greek midwife. Her tried and tested methods became our beacon of light in the sometimes overwhelming world of parenthood.

From the moment we welcomed Leo into this world, Betty's teachings became our roadmap. They guided us through the maze of sleepless nights, diaper blowouts, and endless feeding and cuddles.

Betty's gentle encouragement and unwavering support helped me discover my strength and resilience as a mother. I learned to trust my instincts. I learned to embrace the messy moments. I learned to celebrate the small victories along the way. And as I watched my baby grow and thrive, I couldn't help but marvel at the incredible transformation that had taken place within our little family.

To all the new moms embarking on this adventure, I offer these closing thoughts:

Embrace the journey with an open heart and an open mind. Lean on your support network. It could be a trusted midwife like Betty, fellow moms, or loved ones who offer a listening ear and a comforting shoulder. Remember that it's okay to make mistakes, ask for help, to shed a tear, and to laugh at the chaos that inevitably ensues.

As you navigate the highs and lows of motherhood, know that you are not alone. You are part of a community of superheroes, each with your own unique powers and strengths. Together, we can overcome any obstacle and face any challenge. We can emerge stronger and more resilient than ever before.

So here's to all you expecting moms out there, as you embark on this incredible journey of motherhood. May you embrace the challenges with courage. Celebrate the victories with joy. Always remember that you have the power to go from zero to superhero on this wonderful journey that you are about to embark on.

Love and light

Joanna x